Mediterranean Chicken & Soups

A Delicious Collection of 50 Chicken, Soups & Other Mediterranean Recipes

Marta Jackson

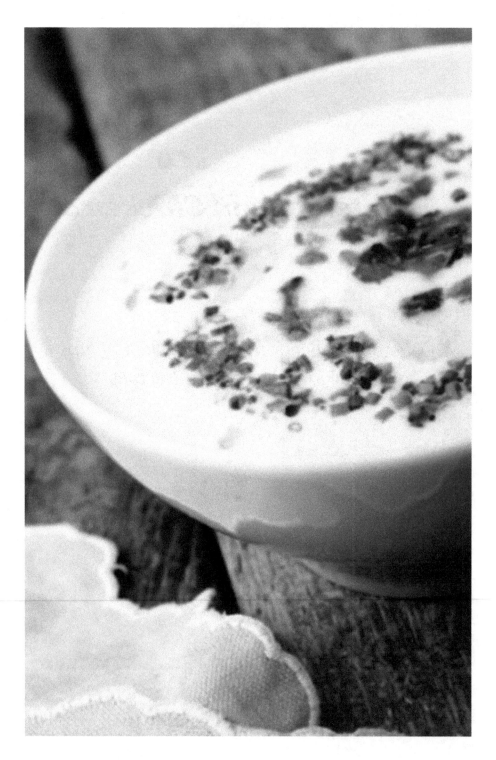

By reading this document, the reader agrees that under no circumstances is the author responsible for any losses, direct or indirect, which are incurred as a result of the use of information contained within this document, including, but not limited to, — errors, omissions, or inaccuracies.

Table of Contents

6

Blackened chicken

Ingredients

- Olive oil
- 1 heaped teaspoon of ground allspice
- 300g of quinoa
- 2 x 200g of skinless chicken breasts
- 2 mixed-color peppers
- 1 fresh red chili
- 4 tablespoons of fat-free yoghurt
- 1 punnet cress
- 100g of baby spinach
- 4 spring onions
- 1 bunch of fresh coriander
- 1 bunch of fresh mint
- 1 large ripe mango
- 2 limes
- 2 tablespoons of extra virgin olive oil
- 1 ripe avocado
- 50g of feta cheese
- 1 heaped teaspoon of smoked paprika

Directions

- Firstly, put the quinoa into the pan and generously cover with boiling water.
- Combine the chili together with the spinach, spring onions, leafy mint, and coriander into the processor, blend until finely chopped.
- Toss the chicken with sea salt, black pepper, the allspice, and paprika on a greaseproof pan.
- Fold over the paper, then flatten the chicken.
- Place into the frying pan with 1 tablespoon of olive oil, turning after 4 minutes.
- Then, add peppers to the frying pan, tossing regularly.
- Drain the quinoa, place on to a serving board.
- Toss with the blended spinach mixture, squeeze over the lime juice.
- Add the extra virgin olive oil, mix and season to taste.
- Sprinkle the mango chunks and cooked peppers over the quinoa.
- Scoop curls of avocado flesh over the salad.

- Slice up the chicken, toss the slices in any juices, then add to the salad.
- Crumble over the feta, scatter over the remaining coriander leaves.
- Serve and enjoy with a dollop of yoghurt.

Pukka yellow curry

Ingredients

- Natural yoghurt
- 2 onions
- 1 teaspoon of tomato puree
- 1 level teaspoon of ground turmeric
- 4 cloves of garlic
- 1 lemon
- 2 teaspoons of curry powder
- 5cm piece of ginger
- 2 yellow peppers
- 1 organic chicken stock cube
- Olive oil
- 1 mug of basmati rice
- 2 fresh red chilies
- ½ a bunch of fresh coriander
- 1 teaspoon of runny honey
- 8 chicken drumsticks
- 1 x 400 g tin of chickpeas

Directions

- Place 1 onion, pepper, garlic, and ginger into a food processor.
- Then, crumble in the stock cube with the chili, coriander stalks, honey, and spices. Blend until paste forms.
- Place a large casserole pan on a medium-high heat.
- Fry the chicken drumsticks with a splash of olive oil for 10 minutes, turning occasionally.
- Remove the chicken to a plate, leaving the pan on the heat.
- Add the remaining onion and pepper to the pan, let cook briefly.
- Then place in the paste, let cook for 5 minutes.
- Pour in 500ml of boiling water.
- Drain the chickpeas, add with the tomato puree and a pinch of sea salt and black pepper, then stir.
- Return the chicken to the pan, cover, simmer gently for 45 minutes over low heat.

- Place in 1 mug of rice with 2 mugs of boiling water into a pan with a pinch of salt let simmer for 12 minutes covered.
- Serve and enjoy.

Roasted chicken breast with lemony Bombay potatoes

Ingredients

- Olive oil
- 200g of potatoes
- A few sprigs of fresh coriander
- 2cm piece of ginger
- ¼ teaspoon of ground turmeric
- ½ red pepper
- 1 free-range chicken breast
- ½ teaspoon of ground cumin
- 1 lemon

Directions

- Preheat the oven to 400°F.
- Cook the potatoes in boiling salted water for 6 minutes, drain and steam dry.
- Add the turmeric, cumin, coriander leaves, ginger, pepper, grate lemon zest to a bowl.
- Squeeze a little juice from the remainder of the lemon into the bowl.

- Shake the potatoes up in the colander, add to the bowl with the chicken.
- Drizzle with olive oil.
- Season with sea salt and black pepper, toss to coat.
- Remove the chicken from the bowl, place the potato mixture into a baking dish.
- Spread out into a single layer topping with the lemon slices, then drape over the chicken.
- Drizzle with olive oil, cook in the middle of the oven for 25 minutes.
- Serve and enjoy.

Chicken and squash cacciatore

Ingredients

- 8 black olives
- 250ml of Chianti
- 1 onion
- 4 chicken thighs, bone in
- 1 leek
- 4 cloves of garlic
- 200g of seeded whole meal bread
- Olive oil
- 2 fresh bay leaves
- 2 sprigs of fresh rosemary
- ½ a butternut squash
- 100g of shell nut mushrooms
- 2 rashers of smoked pancetta
- 2 x 400g tins of plum tomatoes

Directions

- Preheat your oven to 375°F.
- Place a large ovenproof casserole pan on a medium heat.

- Place sliced pancetta, rosemary leaves, 1 tablespoon of olive oil, onion, garlic, bay leaves, and leek in the pan. Stir regularly for 10 minutes.
- Add the stalk with the whole mushrooms, squash to the pan.
- Remove and discard the chicken skin and add the chicken to the pan.
- Pour in the wine, let reduce slightly.
- Add the tomatoes and break them up with a wooden spoon.
- Half-fill each tin with water, swirl about, pour into the pan, mix.
- Destone and poke the olives into the stew.
- Bring to a gentle simmer.
- Transfer to the oven, let cook for 1 hour.
- Season, and adjust accordingly.
- Serve and enjoy.

Barbecued chicken

Ingredients

- 24 ripe cherry tomatoes
- 2 sprigs of fresh rosemary
- Olive oil
- 1 lemon
- 1 teaspoon of wholegrain mustard
- 400g of green beans
- 4 skinless chicken breasts
- Extra virgin olive oil

Directions

- Preheat the oven to 200°F.
- Place rosemary leaves and a pinch of sea salt in a mortar, bash well.
- Add the grated lemon zest and squeeze in half the juice with 2 tablespoons of olive oil.
- Open the chicken breast and flatten
- Pour the rosemary marinade over the chicken, let marinate briefly.
- Mix the mustard with the remaining lemon juice and more extra virgin olive oil.

- Place the tomatoes onto a tray, season, roast for 20 minutes.
- Cook the beans in a pan of boiling salted water for 5 minutes.
- Drain, toss in the mustard dressing, add the roasted tomatoes.
- Preheat a barbecue.
- Barbecue the chicken breasts for 5 minutes, turning regularly.
- Serve and enjoy with beans and tomatoes.

All in one rice and chicken

Ingredients

- 250g of long-grain rice
- Olive oil
- 2 teaspoons of ground coriander
- 1 tablespoon of runny honey
- 2 chicken legs
- A few sprigs of fresh coriander
- 2 chicken thighs
- 1 onion
- 1 clove of garlic
- 1 heaped teaspoon of ground cumin
- 150g of dates

Directions

- Heat a splash of olive oil, then brown the chicken legs and thighs in a pan. Remove.
- Add diced onion, let sweet, then add crushed garlic with the spices in the same a pan.
- Let cook for 2 minutes, stir in the rice together with the dates, honey, and browned chicken.

- Cover with water, let boil, then let simmer, for 30 minutes covered over low heat.
- Season with sea salt and black pepper.
- Scatter over the chopped coriander leaves.
- Serve and enjoy.

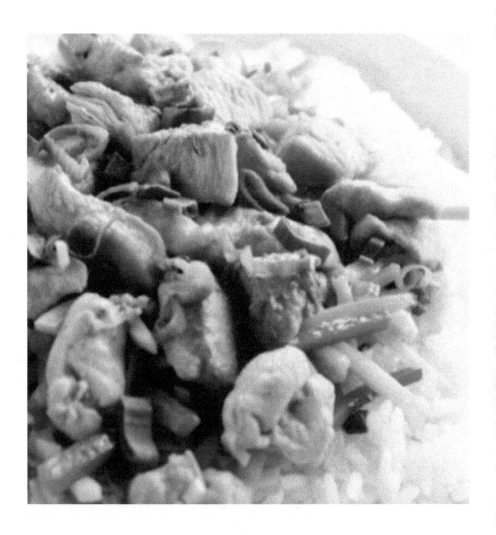

Mediterranean Sea diet soup recipes

Spinach and tortellini soup

Ingredients

- 1 large handful of spinach
- 200g of tortellini
- 1-liter organic chicken
- 2 fresh bay leaves
- 50g of frozen peas

Directions

- Firstly, pour the stock into a large pan.
- Then, add the bay leaves, bring to the boil.
- Add the tortellini, let cook for 4 minutes.
- Add the peas, let cook for a further 3 minutes.
- Add the spinach and cook until wilted.
- Place into bowls.
- Serve and enjoy with crusty bread.

Tortellini in brodo

Ingredients

- 50g of Parmesan cheese
- 150g of beef shank bones
- 75g of prosciutto di Parma
- olive oil
- 1 pinch of ground nutmeg
- 300g of free-range chicken thighs and drumsticks
- ½ of an onion
- 50g of mortadella di Bologna
- 1 stick of celery
- 1 carrot
- 200g tipo flour
- 300g of beef brisket
- 2 large free-range eggs
- 75g pf lean minced beef

Directions

- Add carrots, chicken, unpeeled onion, celery, and a pinch of salt to a stockpot, cover with enough water.

- Bring to boil, then cover, let simmer for 4 hours as you skim occasionally.
- Blend the tipo flour with eggs in a food processor until soft but firm dough, wrap in Clingfilm, let rest for 30 minutes.
- Heat a little olive oil, season the mince and fry until cooked through.
- Drain any water, let cool.
- Transfer to a blender with the prosciutto, mortadella, grated parmesan, and nutmeg. Blend until fine.
- Divide the dough into 8 pieces. Use a pasta machine to roll out 1 piece into a long, flat, thin strip. Slice into 3cm squares.
- Lightly dust a tray with flour.
- Place a ¼ of a teaspoon of filling in the middle of a square of pasta.
- Fold the pasta over into a triangle, and press to seal.
- Repeat until you have used all the rolled-out dough.

- Strain the stock and discard the meat and vegetables.
- Taste and adjust the seasoning accordingly.
- Bring to the boil, add tortellini and cook for about 3 minutes.
- Serve and enjoy.

Summery pea soup with turmeric scallops

Ingredients

- ¼ teaspoon of ground turmeric
- 2 teaspoons of tamarind paste
- 1 bunch of spring onions
- 1 clove of garlic
- 175g of queen scallops
- 5cm piece of ginger
- ½ teaspoon of mustard seeds
- 1 fresh green Bird's-eye chili
- ½ a lime
- 1 teaspoon of cumin seeds
- 10 fresh curry leaves
- Groundnut oil
- 3 fresh curry leaves
- 800ml of organic vegetable
- 450g of fresh or frozen peas
- ½ teaspoon of jiggery

Directions

- Toast the cumin seeds, add 2 tablespoons of oil with the spring onions, garlic, ginger, chili, and curry leaves.
- Fry until sizzling, then pour in the stock and bring to the boil.
- Add the peas, let simmer for 5 minutes.
- Stir in the jiggery with the tamarind paste.
- Season to taste.
- Blender to purée until smooth. Set aside.
- The heat 1 tablespoon of olive oil over a high heat.
- Add the mustard seeds and stir continuously to form soup.
- Mix in the turmeric with the curry leaves, scallops, fry briefly on each side, until beginning to brown.
- Reheat the soup, taste, and adjust.
- Serve and enjoy.

Ham ribollita

Ingredients

- 150g leftover ham
- 300g of cavolo Nero
- 1 onion
- 750ml of organic stock
- 2 cloves of garlic
- 1 x 400g tin of cannellini beans
- 2 sticks of celery
- 1 carrot
- Olive oil
- 2 teaspoons of fennel seeds
- 100g of spinach
- 1 x 400g tin of plum tomatoes

Directions

- Heat a drizzle of olive oil over a medium heat.
- Then, add celery, carrot, onion, garlic, and fennel seeds, and season.
- Cook over low heat for 10 minutes covered, until golden brown, stirring regularly.

- Mash most of the cannellini beans, add to the pan with the liquid from the tin, tomatoes, and the stock.
- Let simmer for more 10 minutes.
- Stir in chopped cavelo Nero, torn ham, and remaining beans, and spinach.
- Simmer until the greens have cooked down.
- Serve and enjoy.

Minestrone soup

Ingredients

- 2 x 400g tins of beans
- 100g of dried pasta
- 4 rashers of smoked streaky bacon
- Olive oil
- Parmesan cheese
- 1 clove of garlic
- 2 small onions
- Extra virgin olive oil
- 1 x 400g tin of quality plum tomatoes
- 2 fresh bay leaves
- 2 carrots
- 2 sticks of celery
- 2 large handfuls of seasonal greens
- 1 vegetable stock cube

Directions

- Heat a large shallow casserole pan on a medium-high heat.
- Sprinkle sliced bacon into the pan with 1 tablespoon of olive oil, stirring occasionally.

- Add the chopped garlic, onion, and bay to the pan when the bacon turns golden.
- Add chopped celery and carrots to the pan.
- Remove and finely chop any tough stalks from your greens and add to the pan.
- Let cook for 15 minutes, stirring regularly.
- Pour in the tinned tomatoes with 1 tin's worth of water.
- Add the beans together with the juice and a pinch of sea salt and black pepper.
- Sprinkle greens into the pan, top with boiling water, then add the pasta.
- Cover, let simmer for 15 minutes.
- Taste, and adjust the seasoning accordingly.
- Serve and enjoy with parmesan cheese.

Spiced parsnips soup

Ingredients

- 800g of parsnips
- 4 sprigs of fresh coriander
- 1 onion
- 4 tablespoons of natural yoghurt
- 2 cloves of garlic
- 1.5 liters of organic vegetable stock
- 5cm piece of ginger
- Olive oil
- 4 uncooked poppadoms
- 1 teaspoon of cumin seeds
- Garam masala
- 200g of red split lentils

Directions

- Start by preheating your oven ready to 350°F.
- Place the parsnips and onions in a large pan over a medium heat with 1 tablespoon of olive oil.
- Cook covered for 20 minutes, stirring occasionally.

- Add the garlic together with the ginger, scatter over the cumin seeds, 1 teaspoon of garam masala and the lentils.
- Cook for 5 more minutes.
- Roughly snap in the uncooked poppadoms, stock, let simmer for 20 minutes.
- Blanch reserved parsnips for 30 seconds in fast boiling water, drain and pat dry.
- Season with sea salt.
- Spread out in a single layer over a couple of oiled baking trays.
- Let roast for 15 minutes.
- Pick over the coriander leaves, sprinkle with a little garam masala, and top with the parsnip crisps.
- Serve and enjoy.

Korean chicken hotpot

Ingredients

- 1 lime
- 150g of shiitake mushrooms
- 2 teaspoons of sesame oil
- 2 teaspoons of Korean chili paste
- 2 large carrots
- 250g of whole wheat noodles
- 1 bunch of spring onions
- 350g of firm silken tofu
- 2 teaspoons of sesame seeds
- 200g of kimchee
- 4 free-range chicken thighs
- 1 liter of organic chicken stock
- 1 teaspoon of low-salt soy sauce

Directions

- Char the mushrooms in a casserole pan on a medium heat for 5 minutes, turning half way.
- Remove the mushrooms to a plate, add the chicken and carrots to the pan.
- Let cook for 10 minutes, stirring regularly.

- Pour in the stock, bring to the boil, let simmer for 20 minutes.
- Stir in the spring onions with mushrooms, tofu, soy sauce, and chili paste.
- Let simmer again for 20 minutes.
- Stir through the kimchee.
- Cook the noodles according to the packet Directions, drain.
- Toss with the sesame oil and seeds.
- Taste the broth, and adjust the seasoning.
- Serve and enjoy.

Playschool tomato soup

Ingredients

- 150g of pasta
- 2 x 400g tins of quality plum tomatoes
- 2 carrots
- 8 slices of sourdough
- 2 leeks
- 2 sticks of celery
- 2 onions
- Extra virgin olive oil
- 125g of mature Cheddar cheese
- 6 large ripe tomatoes
- 4 cloves of garlic
- Olive oil
- 1 organic chicken stock cube
- ½ a bunch of fresh basil

Directions

- Preheat the oven to 375°F.
- Toss all the vegetables and the tomatoes together in a deep roasting tray, season with season well with extra virgin olive oil.

- Spread the vegetables into 1 layer, place in the oven for 40 minutes.
- Bash pickled leaves to a paste, with a pinch of sea salt, until smooth.
- Toss the basil stalks into the roasted vegetable, squeeze the garlic out of its skins into the tray, add tinned tomatoes and stock.
- Bring to a boil over a medium heat.
- Lower the heat, let simmer for about 15 minutes, or until thickened.
- Remove the tray, pulse the soup until smooth.
- Return the soup to the hob over a medium heat.
- Then, season to taste and stir in the pasta.
- Simmer for 5 minutes, or until the pasta is cooked.
- Toast the bread, coarsely grate the cheese.
- Place the hot soup into bowls, scatter over most of the cheese, stir through.
- Top with a piece of toast, scatter over the remaining cheese, and finish with a drizzle of the basil oil.

- Serve and enjoy.

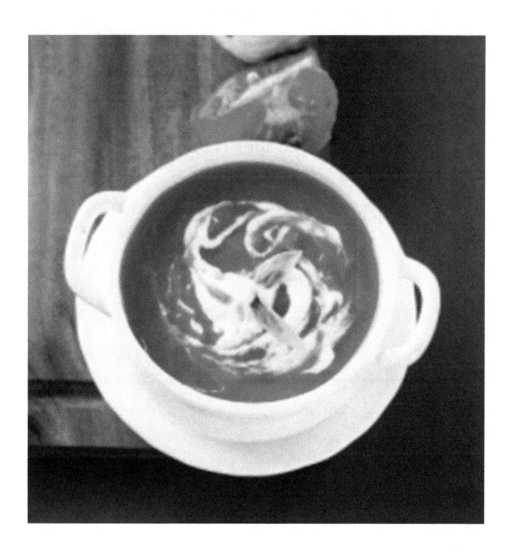

Thai inspired vegetable broth

Ingredients

- 1 teaspoon of fish sauce
- 3 cloves of garlic
- 5cm piece of ginger
- 800ml of clear organic vegetable stock
- 1 small punned shiso cress
- 200g of mixed Asian greens
- 1 lime
- 2 spring onions
- 1 fresh red chili
- 1 teaspoon of soy sauce
- 5 sprigs of fresh Thai basil
- 1 stick of lemongrass
- 2-star anise

Directions

- Bash the lemongrass on a chopping board with a rolling pin until it breaks open.
- Add to a large saucepan together with the garlic, ginger, and star anise.

38

- Pour in the vegetable stock in a pan over a high heat.
- Bring let boil briefly, lower heat and gently simmer for 30 minutes.
- Place in Asian veggies, let cook until they are wilted few minutes to cook time.
- Serve the broth in deep bowls.
- Seasoned with fish sauce and soy sauce, sprinkle with the herbs.
- Serve and enjoy.

Hot and sour chicken broth

Ingredients

- 2 shallots
- 1 large handful of beansprouts
- Fish sauce
- 3 sticks of lemongrass
- 5cm of ginger
- 1.75 liters light organic chicken
- 2 cloves of garlic
- 3 limes
- 2 fresh red chilies
- ½ a bunch of fresh coriander
- Groundnut oil
- 1 bunch of spring onions
- 2 free-range chicken breasts

Directions

- Gently sweat the shallots in a splash of oil until soft.
- Place in the lemongrass together with the ginger, stock, most of the chili and garlic, and fry for 1 minute.

- Add the chicken and simmer for 8 minutes, or until the chicken is cooked through.
- Then, add a splash of fish sauce and squeeze in the lime juice.
- Taste, and adjust seasoning with fish sauce, lime juice or chili.
- Add the coriander, beansprouts, and spring onions.
- Serve and enjoy.

Miso soup with tofu and cabbage

Ingredients

- ½ savoy cabbage
- 100g of silken tofu
- 750ml of organic chicken
- 1 carrot
- 3cm piece of ginger
- Low-salt soy sauce
- 2 cloves of garlic
- 2 tablespoons of miso paste
- 1 fresh red chili

Directions

- Pour the stock into a pan, bring to a boil.
- Add ginger, garlic, and chili to the stock, cover and simmer for 5 minutes.
- Add carrots and cabbage to the pan, cover and simmer for 4 more minutes, or until the cabbage is wilted.
- Then, stir in the miso paste and a good splash of soy sauce to taste.
- Add the tofu and let it stand for a few minutes.

- Serve and enjoy.

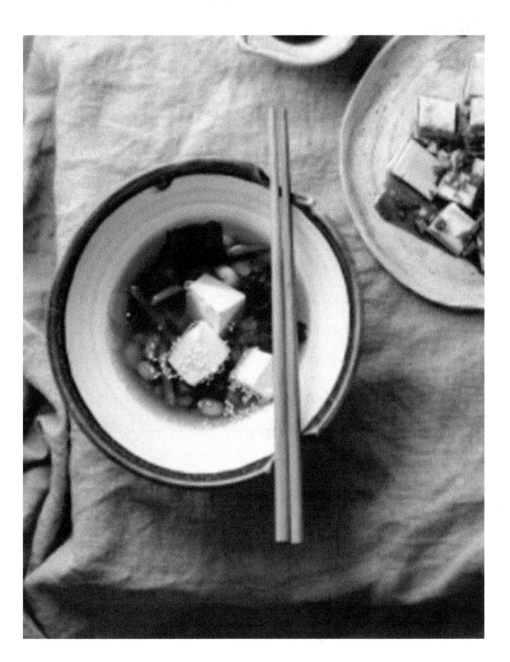

Asian inspired chicken rice balls and broth

Ingredients

- low-salt soy sauce
- 250g of mange tout
- 130g of brown rice
- 1 big bunch of coriander
- 6 spring onions
- 1 handful of beansprouts
- 4 skinless, boneless free-range chicken thighs
- 1 lime
- 2 packets of choi
- 1 stick of lemongrass
- 5cm piece of ginger
- 2 cloves of garlic
- 1 fresh red chili
- 4 kaffir lime leaves
- Sunflower oil
- 8 large raw king prawns
- 2½ tablespoons of miso paste

Directions

- Start by cooking the rice according to the packet Directions.
- Drain any excess water, let cool.
- Place leaves in a food processor with the cooled rice except coriander leaves.
- Add the onion, chicken, lemongrass, ginger, and garlic into the food processor with the kaffir lime leaves, blend until smooth.
- Transfer the mixture onto a board.
- Divide it into 16 pieces and roll each into a ball.
- Place on a plate, chill, covered, until needed.
- Place a large casserole pan over a medium-high heat.
- Add a splash of sunflower oil. Fry the rice balls for 5 minutes, or until golden brown.
- Add prawns to the pan, stir-fry for 1 minute.
- Then, stir in the miso paste with boiling water, let simmer for 10 minutes.
- Add Pak choi cut to 6 pieces with halved mange tout to the pan for the last 2 minutes.
- Stir in the beansprouts for the last 30 seconds.

- Season with a splash of soy sauce.
- Serve and enjoy.

Watercress soup

Ingredients

- 400ml of organic stock
- 2 potatoes
- 3 bunches of watercress
- 2 onions
- Olive oil
- 2 cloves of garlic

Directions

- In a large saucepan, heat bit of olive oil.
- Sauté the potato with onion and garlic until the onions are translucent.
- Add the stock and simmer until the potato is soft.
- Add chopped watercress, let simmer for 4 minutes.
- Liquidize the soup until smooth in a blender.
- Serve and enjoy with a swirl of crème fraiche.

Simple noodle soup

Ingredients

- 300g of ready-prepared rice vermicelli
- 4 spring onions
- 1 splash of soy sauce
- 1 stick of lemongrass
- 2 cloves of garlic
- 225g of raw frozen prawns
- ½ a lime
- 2 fresh red chilies
- A few sprigs of fresh coriander
- 1 liter of organic chicken stock
- 1 bok choy

Directions

- Bring the stock to boil in a large saucepan, lower heat, let simmer.
- Add bok choy, prawns, spring onions, lemon grass, and garlic to the stock.
- Cook for briefly, until the prawns have turned pink and the bok choy has wilted.

- Divide the vermicelli between 4 bowls and ladle over the soup.
- Then, scatter the chili with the coriander on top.
- Season with soy and lime juice.
- Serve and enjoy.

Fish soup

Ingredients

- 400g of prawns
- Olive oil
- 1 small bulb of fennel
- 1 leek
- Extra virgin olive oil
- 1 bunch of fresh thyme
- 3 sticks of celery
- 1 small glass of white wine
- 1 fresh red chili
- 4 cloves of garlic
- 4 tomatoes
- 440g of white fish

Directions

- Begin by gently cooking over medium heat the fennel together with the leek, celery, most of the chili and the garlic in olive oil, until soft.
- Add 1-liter water with the wine.
- let boil, then reduce heat, simmer until vegetables are cooked.

- Add the tomatoes together with the thyme and fish.
- Once the fish turns opaque, add the prawns, let simmer for 2 minutes until prawns are cooked.
- Season to taste.
- Serve and enjoy with a drizzle of extra virgin olive oil and a scattering of fresh chili.

Parsnip, sage, and white bean soup

Ingredients

- 1 parsnip
- 1 onion
- 1 organic liter of chicken stock
- 2 large parsnips
- 2 sprigs of fresh sage
- Olive oil
- 1 x 420g tin of cannellini beans
- 1 sprig of fresh sage
- 1 fresh bay leaf

Directions

- Heat 50ml of olive oil over a medium heat.
- Cook the onion together with parsnips for 10 minutes, or until softened.
- Add the bay leaf together with the beans, sage, and stock.
- Season and let simmer for 15 minutes.
- For the crispy parsnips, preheat the oven to 400°F.

- Brush the parsnip slices and sage leaves with oil.
- Then, bake for 10 minutes, or until crispy.
- Remove and discard the bay leaf from the soup.
- Beat with a stick blender until smooth.
- Taste and adjust the seasoning accordingly.
- Serve and enjoy with a drizzle of olive oil and the parsnip crisps on top.

Pumpkin and ginger soup

Ingredients

- 125ml of coconut milk
- 1kg of pumpkin
- 1-liter organic vegetable stock
- 2 shallots
- ½ tablespoon of chili powder
- 75g of ginger
- A few sprigs of fresh herbs
- Extra virgin olive oil
- 1 lime

Directions

- Put the pumpkin together with the shallots, ginger, and bit of oil in a large saucepan, sauté until soft.
- Add the stock with coconut milk and chili powder.
- Season, bring to the boil, then let simmer for 40 minutes.
- Transfer to a food processor and blend.

- Serve and enjoy with the fresh herbs, lime juice and a splash of coconut milk.

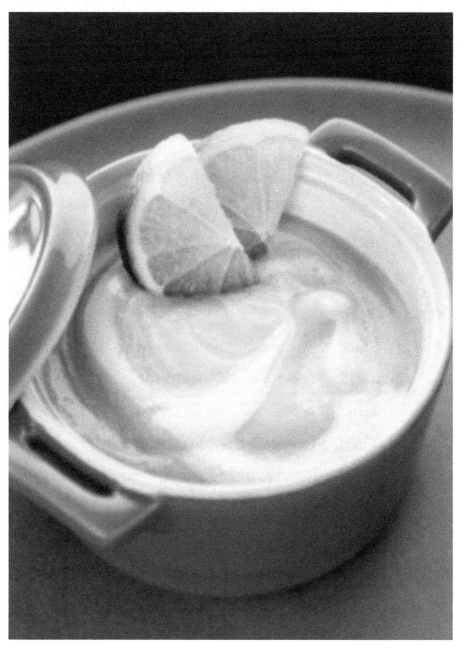

Fresh tomato broth

Ingredients

- 1 x 2kg of whole free-range chicken
- 4 onions
- 20 large ripe mixed-color tomatoes
- 1 tablespoon of tomato purée
- 6 cloves of garlic
- 4 sticks of celery

Directions

- Place the chicken together with the onions, garlic, celery, and tomatoes in a larger saucepan.
- Then, add enough cold water to cover, bring to the boil over a high heat covered for 30 minutes.
- Lower the heat when it begins to boil, let simmer over medium heat with the lid askew for 1 hour, or until the chicken is cooked through.

- Only remove the chicken and put aside.
- Sieve the soup and discard what is trapped.
- Serve and enjoy with a drizzle of basil oil, herbs.

Super tasty miso broth

Ingredients

- 1 x 200g of skinless free-range chicken breast
- 1 handful of colorful curly kale
- 20g of dried porcini mushrooms
- 1 red onion
- 1 sheet of nori
- Groundnut oil
- Rice or white wine vinegar
- 150g of mixed exotic mushrooms
- 1 x 5cm piece of ginger
- 150g of mixed brown and wild rice
- 1 heaped teaspoon miso paste
- 800ml of chicken stock
- 6 radishes

Directions

- Cook as per the package Directions. Drain.
- Rehydrate the porcini in boiling water in a small bowl,

- Place sliced onion, groundnut oil in a medium pan on a medium-high heat.
- Cook briefly until dark golden, stirring occasionally.
- Lower the heat to medium
- Add the ginger with miso paste, porcini with soaking water, and stock.
- Cover and simmer for 20 minutes.
- Toss the radishes in a splash of vinegar with a small pinch of sea salt.
- Stir through sliced chicken, torn kale, nori, broken mushroom.
- Re-cover and cook for 4 minutes. Drain and divide the rice between bowls.
- Season the broth according to your preference.
- Serve and enjoy.

Roast carrot and fennel soup

Ingredients

- ½ teaspoon of dried yeast
- 1kg of carrots
- 250g of strong bread flour
- 1 onion
- 1 teaspoon of fennel seeds
- 1 teaspoon of sugar
- Olive oil
- 2 cloves of garlic
- 1.6 liters of organic vegetable stock
- 2 bulbs of fennel
- 100ml of single cream

Directions

- Preheat your oven to 375°F.
- Place carrots, onion, and fennel in a roasting dish, toss with 2 tablespoons of oil.
- Roast for 20 minutes, add the unpeeled garlic cloves.

- Stir vigorously and return to the oven for further 20 minutes, or until the vegetables are soft.
- Discard garlic cloves.
- Put the roasted vegetables in a large pan with the vegetable stock and bring to the boil.
- Then, Simmer gently for 15 minutes, liquidize with a stick blender, until smooth.
- Toast the fennel seeds in a dry frying pan briefly until fragrant.
- Crush roughly, pour into a bowl with the flour and sea salt.
- Dissolve the yeast and sugar in in hot water.
- Add to the flour mixture with the olive oil and hot water and mix until dough foams, knead.
- Divide the dough into 8 and roughly roll each one into a thin oval.
- Stack them up, separating them with baking paper.
- Heat a griddle pan until it's smoking hot, add the flatbreads.

- Cook for briefly on each side, until charred and puffed up.
- Serve and enjoy.

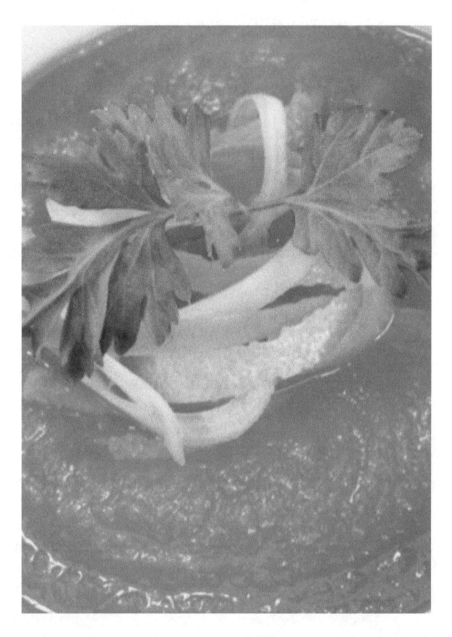

Chicken and vegetables soup

Ingredients

- 1 chicken carcass and bones
- 2 large onions
- 2 sticks of celery
- 1 leek
- Olive oil
- 2 sticks of celery
- 1 bunch of fresh flat-leaf parsley
- 5 black peppercorns
- 4 carrots
- 1 bunch of fresh flat-leaf parsley
- 2 courgette
- 200g of cooked chicken
- 100g of orzo
- 50g of frozen peas

Directions

- Place in a large saucepan quartered onions, with chicken carcass, carrots, celery, peppercorns, and parsley.

- Cover with cold water, season with a little sea salt.
- Bring to the boil over a medium heat, skimming any froth off the surface.
- Lower heat and simmer slowly for 3 hours when covered.
- Strain the broth, let cool.
- Add a splash of oil to a separate large saucepan and place over a medium heat.
- Add onion, leek, celery, carrots, courgette, and parsley. Sauté for 5 minutes.
- Stir in the orzo and stock, bring to a boil.
- Lower the heat and simmer until the veggies are cooked.
- Stir in the peas and chicken until heated through.
- Season to taste.
- Serve and enjoy.

Store cupboard lentil soup

Ingredients

- 1 organic vegetable stock cube
- 2 red onions
- ½ teaspoon dried thyme
- 200g of dried lentils
- Olive oil
- 2 carrots
- 1 x 410 g tin of cannellini beans
- 3 sticks celery
- ½ a dried chili
- 2 cloves garlic
- 6 rashers of smoked streaky bacon
- A few sprigs fresh flat-leaf parsley

Directions

- Heat olive oil over a medium heat
- Add the bacon and fry slowly until crispy, then crumble in the dried chili, dried thyme, carrot, celery, onion, and garlic.
- Cook gently for about 15 minutes covered until all the vegetables are soft.

- Add the lentils with a liter of water.
- Bring to the boil and simmer until the lentils are soft.
- Drain, then place in the cannellini beans.
- Bring back to the boil and simmer for another 10 minutes.
- Season with sea salt and black pepper.
- Add into bowls and drizzle with extra virgin olive oil and the chopped parsley.
- Serve and enjoy.

Ribollita

Ingredients

- 310g of cavelo Nero
- 1 bay leaf
- 2 large handfuls of good-quality stale bread
- 1 ripe tomato
- 1 pinch of dried red chili
- 1 small potato
- Extra virgin olive oil
- 1 x 400g tin of plum tomatoes
- 2 small red onions
- 2 carrots
- 3 cloves of garlic
- 3 sticks of celery
- Olive oil
- 1 pinch of ground fennel seeds

Directions

- Place beans in a pan with bay leaf, tomatoes, and potatoes cook until the beans are tender. Drain and discard the bay leaf, tomato and potato. Reserve some bean water.

- Heat a saucepan with a splash of olive oil.
- Add the vegetables to the pan together with the ground fennel seeds and chili.
- Sweat very slowly on a low heat with the lid just ajar for 20 minutes until soft.
- Add the tomatoes and bring to a gentle simmer briefly.
- Add the cooked and drained beans with a little of the reserved water, bring back to the boil.
- Moisten and stir the bread.
- Continue cooking for about 30 minutes.
- Season with sea salt and black pepper.
- Stir in extra virgin olive oil.
- Serve and enjoy.

Corn chowder soup

Ingredients

- 1 medium potato, peeled and cut into little cubes
- 3 spring onions
- 1 medium onion
- Olive oil
- ½ teaspoon of dried thyme
- ¼ cup of fresh chives, chopped, or parsley
- 1 stalk celery
- 175g of frozen corn
- 1 tablespoon of plain flour
- 840ml of semi-skimmed milk

Directions

- Heat the olive oil in a medium saucepan over a medium heat.
- Add the celery, onion, and thyme.
- Stir until vegetables start to brown.
- Sprinkle the flour over the veggies and stir briefly.

- Pour in the milk, then add the potato let boil, stirring the whole time so the soup, until the potatoes are tender in 10 minutes.
- When the potatoes are tender, stir in the corn together with the spring onion and celery leaves.
- Bring the soup back to the boil.
- Serve and enjoy with crusty brown bread.

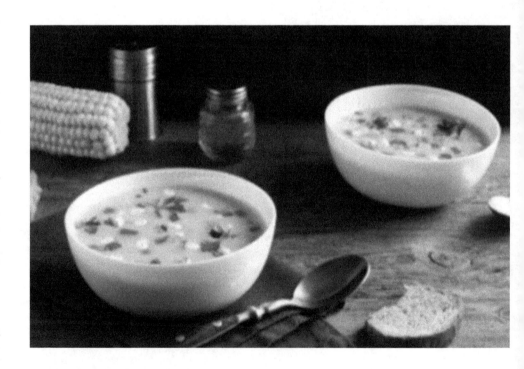

Roasted cauliflower and coconut soup

Ingredients

- 600g of cauliflower
- 1 x 400g tin of reduced-fat coconut milk
- 1 heaped teaspoon of ras el hanout
- 4 cloves of garlic
- 1 heaped teaspoon of ground cinnamon
- 3 tablespoons of chili oil
- Olive oil
- 1 handful of unsweetened coconut flakes
- 2 onions
- 600ml of vegetable stock

Directions

- Preheat your oven to 350°F.
- Place the onions, cauliflower in a roasting tray with the unpeeled garlic cloves and sprinkle with the cinnamon and ras el hanout.
- Season, then drizzle with olive oil.
- Toss, and place into the oven for 30 minutes, or until cooked through.

- Scatter the coconut flakes on to a small tray, place briefly into the oven to toast.
- When the vegetables are ready, remove the garlic cloves and scrape all the vegetables into a large saucepan.
- Squeeze the garlic out of its skins and add to the mixture.
- Pour in the coconut milk with stock, bring to the boil.
- Lower the heat, let simmer for 5 minutes.
- Blend the soup until creamy and smooth, adjust with water if too thick.
- Taste and adjust the seasoning.
- Serve and enjoy topped with the toasted coconut flakes and a drizzle of chili oil.

Chicken noodle soup

Ingredients

- 1 pinch of saffron
- Dry sherry
- Sweet ginger vinegar
- 200g of small carrots
- 100g of baby leeks
- 1 handful of fresh parsley stalks
- 300g of mixed fine pasta shapes
- 2 cloves of garlic
- 2-3 fresh bay leaves
- 200g of small onions
- 1 celery heart
- 5cm of piece of ginger
- 1 x 1.4kg of whole free-range chicken

Directions

- Place celery, carrots, garlic, and onions into a very large saucepan with the chicken, bay leaves, and parsley stalks.
- Season with sea salt and black pepper, then add enough water to cover the chicken.

- Bring to the boil, lower the heat down, let simmer for 1 hour.
- Empty the pan except for stock, then shred the chicken.
- Bring the stock back to the boil and add a good splash of sherry with the saffron and a splash of ginger vinegar.
- Add the pasta and continue to boil until the pasta is al dente.
- Return the chicken and vegetables to the pan and simmer over low heat until warmed through.
- Serve and enjoy.

Clear Asian noodle soup with prawns

Ingredients

- 1 carrot
- 100g of runner beans
- 2 large free-range eggs
- 250g of brown rice noodles
- 200g of cooked peeled king prawns
- 3cm piece of ginger
- 2 fresh hot Thai chilies
- 2 liters of organic chicken stock
- 2 tablespoons of sesame seeds
- 2 tablespoons of low-salt soy sauce
- 6 radishes
- 4 spring onions
- 2 cloves of garlic
- 2-star anise
- 6 cloves

Directions

- Start by cooking the eggs in boiling water for 5 minutes.

- Let cool under cold running water, peel and keep aside.
- Cook the noodles according to the package Directions, drain, leave in a dish of cold water.
- Add ginger and chili to a large pot together with the stock, unpeeled garlic cloves, soy sauce, star anise, and cloves.
- Bring to a simmer, put off the heat, let infuse for 20 minutes.
- Cook runner beans with carrot in a pan of boiling water for 2 minutes.
- Drain, then plunge into cold water.
- Strain the stock into a clean pot, return to a medium heat, then add sliced prawns.
- Cook until just heated through.
- Toast the onions and radishes with the sesame seeds in a dry frying pan.
- Drain the rice noodles and divide between 4 bowls.
- Sit the beans, carrot, and prawns on top.

- Place over the broth and top with the radishes, spring onions, half an egg, and toasted sesame seeds.
- Serve and enjoy.

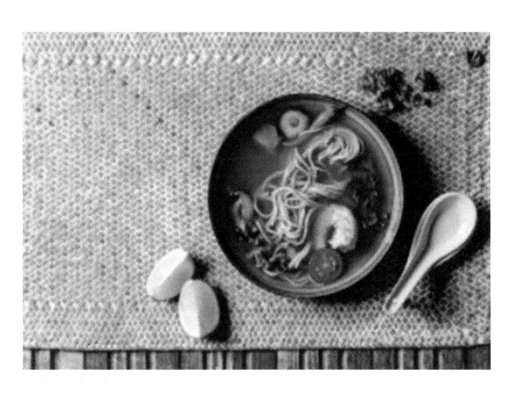

Sweet potato, coconut, and cardamom soup

Ingredients

- 1 pinch of dried chili flakes
- 1 teaspoon of coriander seeds
- 3 green cardamom pods
- 2 jarred roasted peppers
- 800ml of organic vegetable
- 1 onion
- 100g of baby spinach
- 1 x 400ml tin of low-fat coconut milk
- 4cm piece of ginger
- 4 large poppadum
- 600g of sweet potato
- 2 cloves of garlic
- 3 tablespoons of groundnut oil
- 1 lemon

Directions

- Crush the cardamom seeds in a mortar.
- Heat groundnut oil over a low heat, then add the onion with a small pinch of sea salt let cook

for 10 minutes in a large saucepan, stirring often.

- Stir in the sweet potato together with the ginger, garlic, and crushed cardamom seeds.
- Let cook for 2 minutes, then add the coconut milk.
- Allow it to simmer for 2 minutes, stir in the stock.
- Cover with a lid, and leave to simmer gently for 15 minutes.
- Liquidize the soup in a blender until smooth.
- Season with a pinch of salt and black pepper and a squeeze of lemon juice.
- Heat groundnut oil in a frying pan, add crushed coriander seeds and chili flakes.
- Let cook for 1 minute.
- In a dry pan, toast the coconut flakes.
- Add sliced peppers to the spices with the spinach.
- Continue cooking until the spinach has wilted down.
- Season and stir in the toasted coconut flakes.

- Place the soup into bowls
- Serve and enjoy topped with red pepper.

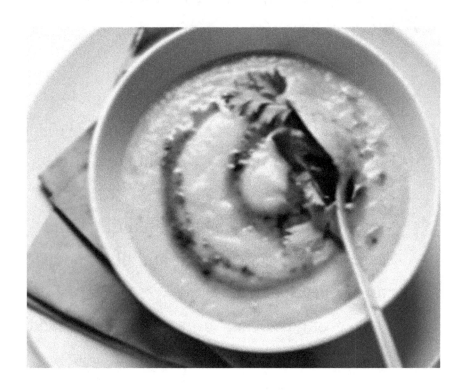

Beetroot and tomato borscht

Ingredients

- 2 celery stalks
- 1 clove of garlic
- 1.2 liters of organic beef stock
- 2 tablespoons of tomato purée
- A few sprigs of fresh dill
- 1 teaspoon of caster sugar
- 1 x 400g tin of plum tomatoes
- 2 large beetroot
- ½ of a small red cabbage
- 2 carrots
- 4 tablespoons of sour cream
- 1 red onion

Directions

- Begin by pouring tomatoes into a large pan, stir in the onion with carrots, celery, garlic, beef stock, beetroot, tomato purée, and sugar.
- Bring to the boil and simmer gently for 5 minutes.

- Add the shredded cabbage, let simmer for another 30 minutes or so.
- Blend the soup until smooth.
- Serve and enjoy hot with swirls of the sour cream, then sprinkled with chopped dill.

Pistou soup

Ingredients

- 6 sprigs of fresh basil
- 60g of Parmesan cheese
- 1 onion
- 1 x 400g tin of borlotti beans
- 8 cloves of garlic
- 3 leeks
- 7 tablespoons of extra virgin olive oil
- 1 x 400g tin of cannellini beans
- 3 potatoes
- 3 carrots
- 1 stick of celery
- 3 courgettes
- 2 sprigs of fresh flat-leaf parsley
- 2 fresh bay leaves
- 250g of baby green beans
- 1 x 400g tin of chopped tomatoes
- 70g of small macaroni

Directions

- Start by heating the olive oil over a medium heat.
- Sauté the onion with garlic and leek for 5 minutes.
- Add the potatoes, carrots, courgette, and celery, bay, green beans and chopped tomatoes.
- Drain and add the beans.
- Cover with water, then season, let simmer until the vegetables are tender.
- Then, add the pasta and simmer until cooked. Regulate water as needed.
- Place garlic, basil leaves, and sea salt in the mortar.
- Pound until puréed, then finely grate in the Parmesan.
- Muddle in the extra virgin olive oil to make a paste.
- Serve and enjoy.

Celeriac and quince soup

Ingredients

- 2 banana shallots
- 1 teaspoon of ground cumin
- 2 cloves of garlic
- olive oil
- A few sprigs of fresh dill
- 1 organic chicken stock cube
- 1 teaspoon of sugar
- 1 quince
- 1 small handful of walnuts
- 1 tablespoon of crème fraiche
- 1 pinch of ground cinnamon
- 1 large celeriac

Directions

- Place olive oil to a large pan, put over a medium-low heat.
- Add the celeriac, shallots, garlic, cumin, cinnamon, sugar, and quince, crumbling in the stock cube.

- Let cook gently for 25 minutes, stirring occasionally.
- Add in enough boiling water to cover the vegetables once all vegetables have softened.
- Uncover and let simmer for 25 minutes, or until the vegetables are cooked through.
- Blend to your preferred consistency.
- Roughly chop the walnuts and toast in a little butter.
- Then, top the soup with a swirl of crème fraiche, a little picked dill and a handful of chopped toasted walnuts.
- Serve and enjoy.

Red lentil, sweet potato, and coconut soup

Ingredients

- ½ a bunch of fresh coriander
- 1 liter of organic vegetable stock
- 750g of sweet potatoes
- 1 x 400g tin of light coconut milk
- 2 red onions
- 125g of red lentils
- ½ tablespoon of cumin seeds
- 1 teaspoon of ground coriander
- Olive oil
- 1 lemon
- 4 cloves of garlic
- 1 fresh red chili

Directions

- Preheat the oven to 350°F.
- Place sweet potatoes with onion wedges in a roasting tray in an even manner.
- Sprinkle over the cumin seeds with ground coriander and a pinch of sea salt and black pepper.

- Then, drizzle with oil, toss to coat.
- Place in the oven for 45 minutes, or until golden.
- Place a large saucepan over a medium-low heat and pour in a lug of oil.
- Sauté the garlic together with the chili and coriander stalks briefly, until lightly golden.
- Add the red lentils to the pan.
- Stir to coat, then pour in the hot stock with coconut milk.
- Raise the heat, let boil, then simmer.
- Cook the lentils for 20 minutes.
- Remove from the oven when veggies are ready, spoon into the pan.
- Add most of the coriander leaves, then blend the soup until creamy with some little texture.
- Taste and adjust the seasoning with lemon juice.
- Serve and enjoy with coriander leaves.

Spiced parsnip and lentil soup with chili oil

Ingredients

- 3 tablespoons of groundnut oil
- 1 small smoked ham hock
- A few sprigs of fresh mint
- 1 onion
- 1 garlic clove
- Fat-free Greek yoghurt
- 3cm piece of ginger
- 400g of parsnips
- Olive oil
- 250g of red lentils
- 2 red chilies
- 2 tablespoons of Rogan paste
- 1.6 liters of organic vegetable stock

Directions

- Soak the ham hock in cold water overnight.
- Drain and place it in a saucepan.
- Cover with cold water, bring it to the boil.
- Lower the heat, let simmer for 2 hours.

- Drain again, and set aside.
- Place the groundnut oil in a pan over a very low heat.
- Add sliced garlic and chilies to the pan, warm for 5 minutes.
- Heat olive oil in a large pan, then add the onion.
- let cook gently for 5 minutes, stirring frequently.
- Add the parsnips together with the rogan paste and ginger, let cook for 5 minutes.
- Add the lentils, stock, and the ham hock, bring to the boil.
- Simmer for about 30 minutes, until the lentils soften.
- Remove and discard the ham bone and liquidize the soup until smooth.
- Return any lean ham to the saucepan and reheat.
- Shred the mint leaves and serve scattered on top of the soup with a dollop of yoghurt.
- Serve and enjoy.

Caldo Verde

Ingredients

- Paprika
- 1 large onion
- Extra virgin olive oil
- 2 cloves of garlic
- 300g of kale
- 150g of chorizo
- 700g of potatoes

Directions

- Start by heating 4 tablespoons of oil in over medium heat.
- Fry the onion with garlic for 5 minutes, or till soft.
- Stir in the potatoes, then season with sea salt, let cook for 5 minutes.
- Add water, then simmer for 20 minutes.
- Then, mash the potatoes into the liquid to produce a smooth purée.
- Add the kale, let simmer for 5 minutes.

- Heat 1 tablespoon of oil in a frying pan over medium heat.
- Fry the chorizo slices, sprinkling with paprika in the pan for 4 minutes.
- Add the chorizo to the soup.
- Place the soup into bowls and season with freshly ground black pepper.
- Serve and enjoy with slices of corn bread.

Baked potato soup

Ingredients

- Sour cream
- 3 large baking potatoes
- 1 Parmesan rind
- 40g of butter
- 1.5 liters of organic chicken
- 1 small bunch of fresh chives
- 1 onion

Directions

- Preheat the oven to 360°F.
- Prick cleaned potatoes with a fork and wrap in foil.
- Place on a rack in the middle of the oven, let cook for about 1 hour 15 minutes.
- Remove, when cool enough, cut into quarters. Let cool completely.
- Melt butter over a medium-low heat, add and cook diced onion for 10 minutes.
- Add the potato with Parmesan rind to the pan.
- Season, and cook for 5 minutes.

- Add the stock, bring to the boil.
- Lower the heat, let simmer for 30 minutes.
- Remove, purée the soup until smooth without the rind.
- Return to the pan.
- Taste, and adjust the seasoning.
- Serve and enjoy with a dollop of sour cream, snipped chives and a pinch of black pepper.

Caprese soup

Ingredients

- 1½ tablespoons red wine vinegar
- 50g of basil leaves
- 1 bulb of garlic
- 4 slices of sourdough bread
- 1kg of mixed tomatoes
- Extra virgin olive oil
- 2 x 125g of balls of buffalo mozzarella
- 4 sun-dried tomatoes in oil
- 1 tablespoon of soft brown sugar

Ingredients

- Preheat the oven ready to 400°F.
- Place cut garlic in a large roasting tray with the tomatoes.
- Drizzle with 1 tablespoon of olive oil.
- Let roast in the oven for 25 minutes, or until the tomatoes have burst.
- Let cool totally.

- Squeeze and roasted garlic into a blender with the roasted tomatoes, sugar, basil, sun-dried tomatoes, vinegar, and 3 tablespoons of oil.
- Blend until smooth, then transfer to a jug.
- Heat a griddle pan and chargrill the sourdough on both sides.
- Serve and enjoy with half a torn mozzarella ball in the center topping with basil leaves and cracked black pepper.

Goulash soup

Ingredients

- 1 tablespoon of tomato purée
- 250g of onions
- 2 cloves of garlic
- ½ tablespoon of caraway seeds
- 200g of potatoes
- 1 green pepper
- 2 tomatoes
- Sour cream
- A few sprigs of fresh marjoram
- Extra virgin olive oil
- 500g of beef shin
- Red wine vinegar
- 1 tablespoon paprika
- 1½ liters of organic beef stock

Directions

- Place a splash of extra olive oil in a large pan.
- Sauté the onions with garlic and pepper until softened.

- Add the beef and continue to cook until the meat is browned and the vegetables are cooked.
- Then, stir in the paprika, let cook for 2 minutes.
- Add the beef stock.
- Bring to the boil until reduced by half.
- Add the marjoram together with the tomatoes, the tomato purée, caraway seeds, a splash of vinegar, season well.
- Add enough stock to cover, let simmer until the meat and vegetables are tender, in 2 hours.
- Add diced potatoes, with the remaining stock.
- Let simmer until the potatoes are cooked.
- Serve and enjoy with a dollop of sour cream.

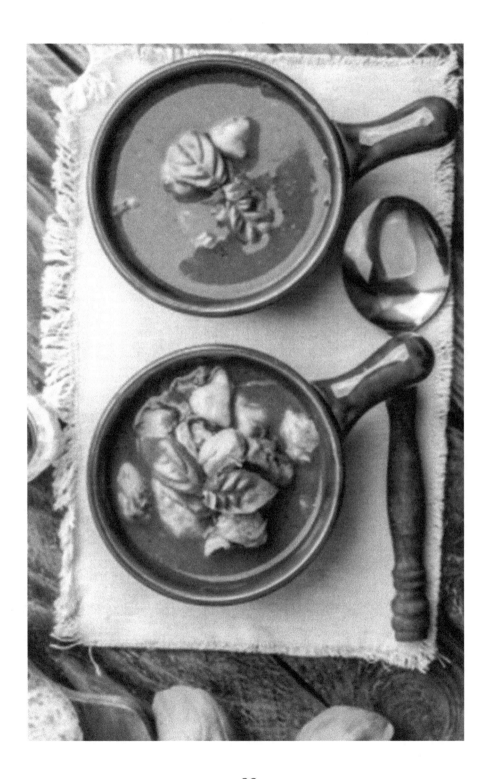

Costa Rican black bean soup

Ingredients

- 4 large free-range eggs
- 3 red onions
- 1 tablespoon of red wine vinegar
- ½ a bunch of fresh thyme
- 2 cloves of garlic
- 2 sticks of celery
- Extra virgin olive oil
- 2 x 400g tins of black beans
- 2 fresh bay leaves
- 1 green pepper
- 4 corn of tortillas
- 1 red pepper
- 2 fresh red chilies
- ½ a bunch of fresh coriander
- Olive oil

Directions

- Drizzle olive oil in a large saucepan over a medium-low heat.

- Add 2/3 of chopped onion, garlic, celery, coriander stalks, and peppers and thyme leaves to the pan.
- Add ½ of chili, gently sauté the veggies for 15 minutes.
- Place black beans with their liquid, bay leaves, and boiling water.
- Raise the heat and bring to the boil.
- Season well.
- Lower the heat, let simmer, for 30 minutes covered, or until creamy.
- Then, crack the eggs directly into the soup over reduced the heat.
- Leave the eggs to poach in the soup for 5 minutes.
- Add chopped coriander with remaining chopped onion, red wine vinegar, and a few tablespoons of extra virgin olive oil. Mix well.
- Serve and enjoy with black bean soup.

Mulligatawny soup

Ingredients

- 1 x 400g tin of chopped tomatoes
- 1 large onion
- 2 cloves of garlic
- 500g leftover of free-range turkey
- 750ml of hot organic chicken
- 1 carrot
- 300g of butternut squash
- 300g of basmati rice
- 1 thumb-sized piece of ginger
- 1 tablespoon of tomato purée
- 1 tablespoon of olive oil
- a few sprigs of fresh coriander
- 1 dried red chili
- 1 tablespoon of curry paste

Directions

- Firstly, heat olive oil in a large saucepan over a medium heat.
- Add the onion together with the garlic, carrot, ginger, and dried chili.

- Cover, and cook, stirring occasionally, until all the vegetables are soft and lightly golden.
- Then, add the butternut squash with tomato purée and curry paste, shred in the turkey, and stir to coat.
- Add the chopped tomatoes.
- Season with sea salt and black pepper.
- Pour in the hot stock and bring to the boil.
- Lower heat and let simmer for 15 minutes.
- Add the basmati rice and simmer for a further 10 minutes.
- Serve and enjoy garnished with coriander leaves.

Turkey and coconut milk soup

Ingredients

- 100g of oyster mushrooms
- 3 Thai shallots
- 200g of cooked, skinless turkey
- 2 bird's-eye chilies
- 1 thumb-sized piece of galangal or ginger
- 3 kaffir lime leaves
- 2 tablespoons of fish sauce
- 3 coriander roots
- A few sprigs of fresh coriander
- 2 lemongrass stalks
- 500 ml organic turkey
- 1 x 400ml tin of light coconut milk
- 1 teaspoon of palm
- 1/2 lime

Directions

- Add the stock with the coconut milk to a large saucepan.
- Bring to the boil, then turn down the heat.

- Add the sugar together with the chilies, lime leaves, lemongrass, shallots, galangal or ginger, and coriander roots.
- Season and simmer gently for 5 minutes.
- Add torn mushroom and shredded turkey to the pan.
- Lower the heat to low.
- Simmer for 3 minutes, and add the fish sauce and lime juice.
- Serve and enjoy hot with some coriander leaves.

Roasted carrot and fennel soup

Ingredients

- ½ teaspoon of dried yeast
- 1 teaspoon of sugar
- 1 teaspoon of fennel seeds
- 1kg of carrots
- 100ml of single cream
- 250g of strong bread flour
- 1 onion
- 2 bulbs of fennel
- Olive oil
- 2 cloves of garlic
- 1.6 liters of organic vegetable stock

Directions

- Preheat the oven to 375°F.
- Place sliced carrots, onion, and fennel in a roasting dish, and toss bit of oil.
- Let roast for 20 minutes, add the unpeeled garlic cloves.
- Stir, return to the oven for 20 more minutes, or until the vegetables are browned.

- Remove, discard the papery skins from the garlic cloves.
- Put the roasted veggies in a large pan with the vegetable stock, bring to the boil.
- Then, simmer for 15 minutes, then liquidize with a stick blender, until completely smooth.
- Toast the fennel seeds in a dry frying pan for 30 seconds.
- Crush roughly with mortar, then pour into a bowl with the flour and sea salt.
- Dissolve the yeast and sugar in hot water.
- Add to the flour mixture with the oil and hot water, mix until dough foams. Knead for 5 minutes.
- Place the dough into an oiled bowl, cover with oiled Clingfilm and set aside to rise.
- Divide the dough into 8, roll each one into a thin oval.
- Stack up, separating them with baking paper.
- Heat a griddle pan until very hot.
- Add the flatbreads let cook briefly on each side, until charred.

- Serve and enjoy with a swirl of cream, a scattering of herby fennel tops.

Apple and celeriac soup

Ingredients

- 200ml of crème fraiche
- 4 tablespoon of olive oil
- 2 onions
- 2 liters of vegetable stock
- A few sage leaves
- 1 celery stalk
- Toasted hazelnuts
- 1 celeriac
- 4 apples
- A few sprigs of thyme

Directions

- Heat half of the olive oil in a large pan.
- Add sliced onions, celery, let cook over a medium heat for 10 minutes until soft.
- Add Chopped celeriac, apples, and thyme leaves to the pan, let cook for 2 to 3 minutes.
- Add the stock and season.
- Let simmer over a low heat for 30 minutes.
- Remove, and blend until smooth.

- Then, stir in half the crème fraiche.
- Heat the remaining olive oil in a pan, fry the sage leaves until crispy.
- Spoon the soup into bowls and top with the remaining crème fraiche.
- Serve and enjoy with a drizzle of extra virgin olive oil, sprinkled with the crispy sage leaves and hazelnuts

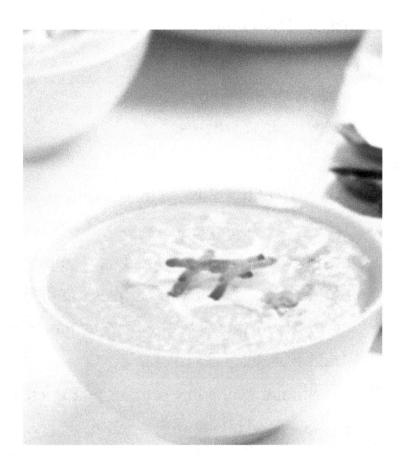

Roasted tomatoes and bread soup

Ingredients

- 2kg of ripe tomatoes
- ½ a bulb of garlic
- 2 red onions
- 1 pinch of dried oregano
- Olive oil
- 1 liter of organic vegetable stock
- A few sprigs of fresh basil
- 1 x 280g of ciabatta loaf
- Red wine vinegar
- Extra virgin olive oil

Directions

- Preheat the oven to 400°F.
- Place cut tomatoes on a large roasting tray.
- Scatter garlic bulbs and wedges of onions into the tray.
- Sprinkle with oregano.
- Season with sea salt and black pepper.
- Drizzle with oil, then let roast for 1 hour, or until the tomatoes sticky.

- Pour in the stock, roughly chop and add the basil stalks with most of the leaves.
- Tear 1 half of ciabatta loaf into the soup.
- Bring to the boil, simmer for 10 minutes.
- Heat a griddle pan to high.
- Slice the remaining ciabatta and griddle until lightly charred on both sides.
- Add 1 splash of red wine vinegar to the soup.
- Blend until fairly smooth.
- Ladle into bowls, drizzle with extra virgin olive oil and scatter with the remaining basil leaves.
- Serve and enjoy with griddled ciabatta on the side.

CPSIA information can be obtained
at www.ICGtesting.com
Printed in the USA
BVHW061252020621
608627BV00008B/606